CHANGE
YOUR STORY
CHANGE
YOUR BRAIN

CHANGE
YOUR STORY
CHANGE
YOUR BRAIN

DR. LINDA MILES

To order additional copies of this book, contact:
Xlibris
1-888-795-4274
www.Xlibris.com
Orders@Xlibris.com
746910

TABLE OF CONTENTS

Mindfulness as the Road to Recovery

Mindfulness as a Path of Self-Discovery

DEDICATION

To Robert, my husband and love.

ACKNOWLEDGEMENTS

Thanks to my dear, life-long friend Lucy Baney, who helped shape and edit this material. Thanks also to my editors Angela Panayotopulos and Christina Morfeld… two of the best.

INTRODUCTION: WHY MINDFULNESS?

"There is nothing noble about suffering except
the love and forgiveness with which we meet
it." -Stephen Levine

In the fast-paced world which we live in, it's easy for the little things to get trampled by the big things. The "little things" as we tend to call them, however, are actually the big things. Peace, positivity, joy, and gratitude: things that are so often underrated and neglected, things that can seem ephemeral or "belonging to other people". And yet these exact things are the essence of life.

Please take a moment to consider the following questions.

- Are you dealing with a medical condition? Yes ☒ No ☐

- Do you feel overwhelmed by situations at home or at work? Yes ☐ No ☒

- Do you find yourself focusing on the negative? Yes ☒ No ☐

- Do you frequently obsess over the past? Yes ☐ No ☒

- Do you anger quickly and/or say things you later regret? Yes ☐ No ☒

- Do you let minor hassles ruin your day?   Yes ☐   No ☒

- Are you having issues interacting with a difficult person?   Yes ☐   No ☒

- Do you worry too much?   Yes ☒   No ☐

- Do you feel that you've lost your mojo, your joy of life?   Yes ☒   No ☐

- Do you suffer from depression, panic, or anxiety?   Yes ☒   No ☐

- Do you wish you were better at "living in the moment"?   Yes ☒   No ☐

- Do you rely on drugs or alcohol to become social or to "escape"?   Yes ☐   No ☒

- Do you feel as if life is passing you by?   Yes ☒   No ☐

Chances are, like most of us, you've answered "yes" to at least one of the above questions. It's not enough that we are bombarded by the world. We are bombarded by our own negative thoughts, rendering ourselves our greatest enemy instead of our best and most long-lasting friend. We might find ourselves trapped in a self-made prison of blame and judgment that prevents us from relishing the good in our lives. We can find ourselves slipping into a downward spiral of self-fulfilling toxic prophecies.

We forget that we have wings and capes to break free of these mind traps and rise above them. We forget that humans have lifted 3,000 pound cars, they've walked on tightropes across Niagara Falls and tread across paths of burning embers, they've literally carved roads through mountains, and they've survived wars and torture chambers only to emerge stronger and more human than ever before. We forget our minds are the most powerful weapon.

Literature helps to remind us. Mindfulness gives us skills to cope.

"Now is where love breathes." -Rumi

THE SCIENCE OF MINDFULNESS

Mindfulness is a scientific approach to acceptance and inner peace, extensively studied by John Kabat-Zinn, Ph.D., at the University of Massachusetts. He defines mindfulness as "paying attention in a particular way; on purpose, in the present moment, and non-judgmentally." In short, mindfulness translates to an enriched awareness of the present.

Dr. Kabat-Zinn's research propelled mindfulness as a way to reduce the pain of patients who dealt with medical illnesses, and as a way to help people tackle everyday life challenges. His work has contributed significantly to a growing movement of mindfulness in areas of medicine, psychology, healthcare, neuroscience, education, corporations, prisons, governmental organizations, and professional sports.

As a psychotherapist, practicing mindfulness is a huge part of my own job description; as a human, practicing mindfulness is my right and my blessing. I've acknowledged mindfulness as the valuable practice that it is and I help others cultivate it within themselves. I've watched firsthand as it has contributed immensely to the lives of many.

However our ancestors termed it, mindfulness has always been a way of life; it's one of the most ancient practices. It's as simple (and simultaneously, as profound) as rediscovering the blessing of freely breathing, the sensation of a caress or a kiss, the vastness of the universe. Happiness can be a benefit of mindfulness. Science shows that happiness has a biological basis; research proves that we can take steps toward creating a positive and healthy mental space for ourselves, despite the stresses of thriving in a demanding and technology-driven world.

By actively exercising kindness and appreciation, we can prompt the brain's natural production of oxytocin and dopamine—two chemicals that enable us to feel pleasure and well-being. In doing so, we simultaneously decrease the secretion of the chemicals adrenaline and cortisol; these chemicals can make us feel stressed and agitated. Though they also serve a purpose—adrenaline is what gives you the extra burst of energy to run away from a crocodile or a mugger, for instance—these can be lethal in long and continuous doses.

"The mind is a wonderful servant, but a terrible master." –Robin S. Sharma

AN EDUCATION IN MINDFULNESS

Best of all, perhaps, is the fact that mindfulness can be learned and mastered. As neuroscientist Dr. Wayne Drevets attests, "In the brain, practice makes permanent." Mindfulness is a lifestyle.

This is wonderful news! While you may need to work at it initially, mindfulness will come more easily and naturally to you over time—and you will discover that the benefits are worth the effort. Focusing on simple pleasures and the present moment is a process that helps us get out of our own heads and into the world around us. This, in turn, allows us to enjoy an increased awareness and connectivity to the blessings and positivity in our lives.

I'm excited you're here with me. Within the pages of this book, I share with you a collection of essays and practices, providing specific examples of how mindfulness can be practiced and the ways in which it can influence positive outcomes in your everyday life. You needn't read it in one sitting. You needn't read it in order. This book is here as a friend, as a quiet yet uplifting conversation. Feel free to come back to whatever chapters apply to your situation at any time, to gain courage and insight from the information within. Unleash your inner power, your humanity. Seize control of your mind and your life. I want you to realize and remember that, ultimately, the magic is in you.

Wishing you joy and mindful awareness,

Dr. Linda Miles

MINDFULNESS AS A SURVIVAL STRATEGY

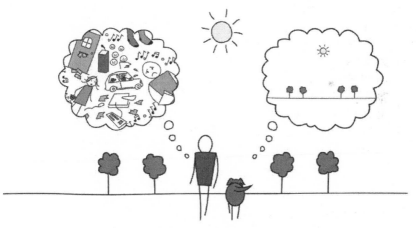

Mind Full, or Mindful?

WHERE DO YOU PUT THE PAIN? A POWERFUL REPERCEPTION OF GRIEF

☑ *Do you feel numbed or overwhelmed with pain?*

☑ *Are you wondering how to deal with loss or grief? Do you find it difficult to imagine how to cope with painful and negative emotions?*

☑ *Are you afraid of facing your pain or grief, for fear of being swallowed by your suffering?*

AN EMPATHETIC DEATH

There are a number of stories, as quiet and as brilliant as gemstones peeking from the ground, that deal with the momentous theme of mortality, the meaning of life, and the meaning of death. Some of the most powerful and poignant of these are actually children's books. One such riveting tale was written by Danish author Glenn Ringtved, illustrated by Charlotte Pardi, and translated to English by Robert Moulthrop. It is stirringly entitled: *Cry, Heart, But Never Break.*

The story tells of Death's house call to four small children who live with their grandmother, whom they love very much and who is dying. In the

1

story, Death is portrayed as a remarkably tender and empathetic character, who leaves his scythe at the door so as to not frighten the children. He compassionately accepts their invitation for coffee because the children believe that this will delay and deter him from his mission, and he even seems genuinely heartbroken by the duty he must do. To brace them for the reality of their grandmother's impending departure, Death shares a story with the four children, trying to give them hope by revealing a different way of seeing things. Death's story is about two brothers—named Sorrow and Grief—who lived in a dark valley and "never saw through the shadows on the tops of the hills"… until they met and fell in love with two sisters, aptly named Joy and Delight.

Perfectly balanced, with the respective boys and girls completing each other, these two couples reenact the theme of essential balance in the universe: day and night, health and sickness, sun and rain, life and death, and so forth. This narrative is Death's way of gently reminding the children that death itself—oxymoronically or not—helps us appreciate and enjoy life. It is a cycle and a balance. When the children head upstairs and realize their grandmother has died, Death whispers: "Cry, heart, but never break. Let your tears of grief and sadness help begin new life."

"Pity arises from meeting pain with fear.
Compassion arises when you meet it with
love." -Anonymous

NOW

Apart from depicting the balance of life and death, *Cry, Heart, But Never Break* subtly illustrates the power of human perception in dealing with and overcoming loss and grief. This can also be described by the idea of "sacred spaciousness", which is a term that grief therapist Stephen Levine uses to describe how he copes with his grieving or terminally ill patients. Pediatrician Amy-Lee Bredlau has also explored this concept in her article entitled "Where Do You Put the Pain?", where she recalls the heartbreaking cases of her child patients who were facing death.

The steps of the NOW approach parallel Dr. Bredlau's journey of self-discovery and her revelation of how to deal with loss.

✧ Notice.

A colleague who trained with Dr. Bredlau once asked her, "Where do you put the pain?" This doctor, like Dr. Bredlau, had noticed that the pain of dealing with dying children affected her deeply and heavily. Finding a way to deal with all this emotion was essential as a doctor and as a human being.

✧ Opportunities.

Asking the question allowed the young doctor to find answers, and exposed her to Dr. Bredlau's strategy: her way of dealing with the pain of being a pediatrician to very sick and dying children was by visiting the child in his or her family home. There she'd watch the child and the siblings running in the grass and enjoying the blessings of nature and familial love, and she'd pinpoint scenes and moments that reminded her that life and joy still surrounded her even in the darkest hours. She also let herself be inspired by the parents' bravery and in the ways that some families simply made the best of their situation.

✧ Within.

Dr. Bredlau chose to see the question—*where do you put the pain?*—as an opportunity to become curious and delve within herself to search for answers. She was able to determine what she needed in order to cope and to thrive, and then found a way to make those house calls to help her cultivate her sacred spaciousness.

> "The deeper that sorrow carves into your being,
> the more joy you can contain." –Khalil Gibran

THE PATH TO MINDFULNESS

In a nutshell, "sacred spaciousness" means that you make room for the pain—as well as for the other emotions that will similarly flow in once you open the floodgates of your heart. Sacred spaciousness means that you do not deny the pain. You create space within yourself for all the emotions, yet then you choose to focus on those which bring you joy and peace. You drink in all the goodness of all the blessings: giving thanks for the humans who are alive, for the sun, for the rain, for the traits of bravery and integrity and generosity that exist in the world around you, and so forth. You are able to sit with the pain, to let it wash over you before it inevitably ebbs away, coming and going as naturally as a wave.

Just as in Death's story described in the Danish storybook, Dr. Bredlau discovered that joy and delight exist alongside sorrow and grief, and it is impossible to fully appreciate or fully conceive of any of these concepts and emotions without contrasting them against their counterparts.

PRACTICE

As a psychotherapist, I strive to help patients embrace both the shadow and the light in their lives. I strive to help them learn to face pain without losing themselves in the suffering. I have found that allowing pain to flow through us in waves is what enables us to make room for sacred spaciousness. It is by facing and acknowledging our grief that we unlock ways to overcome it.

You can practice sacred spaciousness by allowing yourself to first become aware of something that pains you—either a current situation, a gut-wrenching worry, or a heartbreaking memory. Notice how much space those negative feelings occupy in your consciousness as you go through a given day. Now mentally visualize yourself entering your body and moving around the emotions. Handle them gently but firmly, as you would delicate parcels. Create a sanctuary of sacred spaciousness in your mind, and allow the pain to float there along with the myriad of blessings that surround you. Realize all that you have to be grateful for right now and fill this mental space with gratitude.

Remember that even the most painful situations can be dealt with if we learn how to respect the pain, perceive the issue, and balance all of it mentally. Dr. Bredlau deliberately focused on the blessings that existed in the families who cared for a terminally ill child. Like the doctor, we can make room in our minds to fit both the tragedy and the celebration of life. We won't be the first humans who overcome grief and pain, nor will we be the last. But we must soften and soothe our hearts with the balm of blessings to counter the inevitable hurts. Remember Death's advice in the Danish storybook: "Cry, heart, but never break. Let your tears of grief and sadness help begin new life." Cultivate your mind and heart to make room for both sorrow and renewal.

"It is the same with life and death... what would life be worth if there were no death? Who would enjoy the sun if it never rained? Who would yearn for the day if there were no night?" *—Cry, Heart, But Never Break*

FREEDOM FROM MENTAL CAPTIVITY: LESSONS FROM A CONCENTRATION CAMP PRISONER

☑ *Do you find that your thoughts make you more anxious and depressed?*

☑ *Do you have trouble quieting your mind and falling asleep?*

☑ *Is it difficult for you to control your negative emotions?*

SURVIVOR

World-renowned author and psychotherapist Viktor Frankl was a concentration camp prisoner during WWII. He tells his story within the pages of his aptly-titled book, *Man's Search for Meaning,* along with some truly grounding insight. He is not alone—there are many men and women who have emerged from a personal tragedy with their humanity preserved—and yet he speaks up to emphasize a very important message: you must guard your inner life resilience.

No one can make you a prisoner of your own mind unless you let them. You have the power to rewire your brain and choose the alchemy of your own brain chemicals. In this sense, you will always be free.

Despite the degradation, deprivation, and nightmarish misery of the Nazi concentration camp, Frankl clung to his one and most important freedom—the freedom to control his inner life. He realized that, though the Nazis could subjugate him and his fellow prisoners, though they could beat him until his bones cracked and his body numbed, though they could starve him and unclothe him and physically mutilate him, no one could enter his mind without his consent. They could not dehumanize his inner existence. They had no ownership over his mind, heart, or soul.

Frankl made a decision, consciously, to focus on the love he felt for his beloved wife:

"We stumbled on in the darkness, over big stones and three large puddles, along the one road running through the camp. The accompanying guards kept shouting at us and driving us with the butts of their rifles. Hardly a word was spoken; the icy wind did not encourage talk [...] My mind clung to my wife's image, imagining it with uncanny acuteness [...] I understood how a man who has nothing left in this world may still know bliss, be it only for a brief moment, in the contemplation of his beloved. In a position of utter desolation, when a man cannot express himself in positive action, when his only achievement may consist in enduring his sufferings the right way—an honorable way [...] can, through loving contemplation of the image he carried of his beloved, achieve fulfillment."

"Strength does not come from physical capacity.
It comes from an indomitable will." –Mohandas
Gandhi

NOW

There may come an instant in your life when things appear to have gone horribly, horribly wrong. That is life though; without the downs, it'd be impossible to genuinely appreciate the ups—such is human nature. The human range of emotion is spectacular in its extent—if you stop to think about it, it's fascinating that we have the capacity and capability to reach the depths of despair, the heights of ecstasy, the warmth of bliss, the chill of terror, the serenity of peace, and all those myriads of feelings in between. What's even more incredible is the realization—which not all people make—that life is not primarily what happens to you, but how you react to it.

Make something of your life *now*...

⬥ Notice.

Look around and you'll find hundreds of living, breathing examples (and countless more, before our time). A person's sufferings can make or break them—because those are the moments when choices are made. Notice your inner world. What is happening within?

⬥ Opportunities.

Challenges can be obstacles or stepping stones, depending on your perspective. That is when people decide to either fall and fester or fight and flourish. They make a choice, over and over again, about whether their troubles are obstacles or opportunities.

⬥ Within.

How consciously that choice is made relies on the person, and therein lies the power of perception. Realize that no one can alter your inner world without your consent.

THE PATH OF MINDFULNESS

Exile. Abuse. Wars. Toxic relationships. Disaster wreckages. Prisons. Torture chambers. There are people who get out alive—and they all have something in common. They have a burning desire to survive.

It works because they have aligned themselves with a purpose greater than themselves. Always this is an extremely deep emotion—the desire to return to a loved one, the need to persevere and exact revenge for a wronged loved one, the yearning to break free and prove to yourself and to everyone else that you can. There is something beautiful and positive inside these survivors that burns so brightly, so fiercely, that they can't choose to give up. The strongest and most long-lasting of these emotions? The most positive, enduring, powerful quality of all time: love.

> "I survived because the fire inside me burned brighter than the fire around me." –Joshua Graham

Mindfulness is a practice that circles back to love. It's about filtering through the thoughts in our mind and focusing on what we ultimately wish to keep. Our brain is an incredible memory bank, storing positive and negative thoughts. These thoughts have immense power, since they literally affect our body's chemistry. By focusing on negative thoughts or caustic memories, our body generates cortisol and adrenaline—stress signals that cause tension, anxiety, and super vigilance. These chemicals are essential for short-term fight-or-flight scenarios, but are detrimental—even lethal—when experienced constantly for a long period of time. Focusing on positive thoughts, on the other hand, releases feel-good chemicals like dopamine and oxytocin which help us feel mellow, centered, and happy. Such chemicals enable people like Frankl to survive horrific conditions; he had the presence of mind to preserve his strength and will to live, and his purpose and love were the fuel that kept him alive.

PRACTICE

Mindfulness is something you can do anytime, anywhere. It only takes a moment to begin. With the following technique, you will instantly discover how your thoughts alter your body chemistry, and the power you have to control all of this.

→ Close your eyes and recall a time you had a very negative interaction with another person. Look back and really live this memory again, and let yourself feel those destressing emotions. Now open your eyes. How do you feel? Most people report an automatic reaction of increased tension; it's obvious from their clenched teeth or hands, a pressure in their chest or stomach, and increased muscle tightness. If you feel this, it means your body has just unleashed a surge of adrenaline and cortisol.

→ Now close your eyes and recall a time when you felt very close to someone, very loved and cherished. Recall how serene and blissful you felt. Perhaps this is your favorite memory. Now open your eyes and notice how you feel. See the difference? Most people express greater feelings of relaxation, safety, and peacefulness. If you feel these things, it means you've allowed yourself to recall and feel those positive emotions, and your body has secreted oxytocin and dopamine.

Knowing this, you can master the technique so as to center yourself and protect your wellbeing and inner world. During challenging times, you can remember the details of a loving memory and deliberately prompt your body to create positive chemicals that will enhance your calm state of being and your clarity of thought. It can help to perform some sort of ritual—for example, tap on your knees a total of six times as you recall a loving connection, or take six deep breaths. You're linking an action with a thought; next time you can't bring yourself to concentrate, taping six times on your knees may help trigger the memory and thus the happy feelings. Now you also understand why you feel so awful when you relive negative thoughts inside your mind; above all, when you are refraining from nasty thoughts, you are not just being kind to others, you are foremost being kind to yourself and your own health.

"Be not afraid of life. Believe that life is worth living, and your belief will help create the fact." –William James

LABELING THOUGHTS TO ENABLE CLEAR THINKING

☑ *Do you beat yourself up when you fail at something?*

☑ *Does fear stop you from trying again once you've already failed?*

☑ *Do you suffer from the self-abuse of harsh self-judgment?*

WORD POWER

Maya Angelou wrote an essay about the day she lost her first job at sixteen years old. She describes the way she dressed up and landed a job at a fast food restaurant. Unfortunately, her tenure was short-lived; after a brief stint, she was fired. Her mother returned home that day to find Maya on her bed, crying hysterically. Once she'd understood what had happened, her mother countered Maya's tears with her own tough love encouragement: *"Fired? Fired? What.. is that? Nothing. Tomorrow you'll go looking for another job. That's all."*

Maya's mother handled the situation brilliantly by offering Maya a different point of view. She pointed out that "fired" is just a word. Words are merely words, and they have no power but that which we give to them. Maya couldn't see past the word "fired" until her mother taught her to step back and look beyond it—and then to go back out and look for another job.

A word is bundled within a thick layering of assumptions. By noticing what words we focus on—and guiding ourselves to see this with compassionate, nonjudgmental awareness—we can step back and study our assumptions. We can strip them away to reveal the essence of a situation. That is the most effective way of dealing with stress. This is called mindfulness.

> "If I am not good to myself, how can I expect anyone else to be good to me?" –Maya Angelou

NOW

Just like Maya Angelou, we can learn to use the NOW methodology to give ourselves the breathing space we need in order to assess a situation and make our next move:

✧ Notice.

With her mother's encouragement, Maya was able to stop beating herself up and instead think about the harsh connotations she personally applied to words like "fired" and "failure", and the ensuing self-judgment and criticism that erupted from these.

✧ Opportunities.

She then realized that she had the opportunity to rewrite the way she spoke to herself. If we stop to think about it, most of us would immediately realize that our self-talk is extremely negative and critical—we tend to speak to ourselves in a manner that we'd never use with a friend! With a friend we are empathetic, compassionate, considerate, and soothing. But how can we truly extend this compassionate help if we fail to nurture our own selves with these emotions?

✧ Within.

By noticing her inner dialogue, Maya seized the chance to change her thinking and, subsequently, her choices. And this works because our outward behavior always projects, to some level, our inner thought. If we want to create any sort of change, we must begin from within.

THE PATH TO MINDFULNESS

Research shows that those who deal best with stress are characterized by a trait that can be universally cultivated: resilience. These people do not marinate in negative words and harsh judgment. Philippe Goldin, director of the Clinically Applied Affective Neuroscience Project in the Department of Psychology at Stanford University, works with people who suffer from a constant onslaught of negative thoughts and emotions.

Goldin's research reveals that mindfulness meditation greatly affects the way in which the brain responds to negative thoughts. After merely eight weeks of mindfulness training, the participants show significantly increased activity in the brain network associated with processing information when they reflect on negative self-inflicted statements. By paying more attention to the words they say to themselves—and effectively dealing with their reactions to them—they report far less worry and anxiety.

> "Words are seeds that do more than blow around. They land in our hearts and not the ground. Be careful what you plant and careful what you say. You might have to eat what you planted one day." –Anonymous

According to Goldin, mindfulness teaches people how to handle distressing thoughts. By labeling thoughts without judgment, we are able to detach from distressing emotions and see the bigger picture with a clearer mind. Brain scans indicate that the ability to witness thoughts without self-judgment leads to long-term positive changes in the brain—even *as little as ten minutes* a day of mindful meditation has shown immense benefits!

Like Maya, we need to look out for and label the moments when we overgeneralize. She initially thought of *being fired* as a permanent label instead of a temporary situation and a learning experience. It is important to observe negative thoughts, as this helps us begin to question the validity of these "all or nothing" labels. Instead of dramatically criticizing yourself and overgeneralizing a situation—"I'm a failure" or "I'm stupid"—learn to step back and see the situation for what it really is: "I failed at this, but

13

I'll try harder next time to succeed; just the mere fact that I'm not giving up makes me anything but a failure" or "I may have acted stupidly in this situation, but this doesn't make me a stupid person; I have learned how to improve my response next time this happens".

PRACTICE

Neuroscientist Wayne Drevets observes that, in the brain, practice makes permanent. Thus, the more often you practice non-judgmental analysis of and detachment from your own thoughts, the stronger the ensuing connections in your brain. Noting and removing judgmental labels enables you to take positive action.

→ Pay attention to your present thoughts. Allow your thoughts to float around in your mind. Understand that your thoughts and emotions are ephemeral. They will come and go and will always pass through; they need not define you.

→ Take a moment to frame a negative thought. Visualize it however you want, but place it inside something: a bubble (like in the cartoons), a boat, or a box.

→ Label the thought for what it is: an overgeneralization, an overreaction, a very harsh critique, a fear that stems from a past failure, etc.

→ Now that you've labeled it, you can detach yourself from it. You see that the thought is not YOU. Let go of the box, the boat, or the bubble. Mentally watch that thought float away from you. Let it go.

Remember, regardless of the scenario, there are only two possible outcomes: sometimes you'll *win*; sometimes you'll *learn*. Coach yourself in this mentality; first be mindful of what you think, and you will then be able to master your actions and reactions.

"Your beliefs become your thoughts; your thoughts become your words; your words become your actions; your actions become your habits; your habits become your values; your values become your destiny." –Mahatma Gandhi

EVERYDAY MIRACLES: LESSONS FROM THE SNOW CHILD

☑ *Do you spend too much of your life trapped in the past or the future?*

☑ *Are you able to hold the present moment before it slips through your fingers?*

☑ *Do you experience gratitude for everyday indications that you are alive and well?*

BELIEVER

In her touching novel *The Snow Child*, Eowyn Ivey explores universal themes of love, loss, faith, and gratitude. She tells the poignant story of a middle-aged couple (Jack and Mabel), torn by their grief after losing a baby and despairing that they'll never have a family, who move to Alaska for a fresh start. The harsh yet exquisite beauty of the raw Alaskan wilderness inspires them to cherish moments as they rediscover the magnificence and everyday miracles of life.

In one of the book's most quiet yet memorable scenes, Mabel pauses to appreciate a moment as she expresses her gratitude for life's "miracles". She likens "the present" to a snowflake, given its intangibility, temporary nature, and exceptional beauty: "she could not fathom the hexagonal miracle of snowflakes formed from clouds, crystallized fern and feather that tumble down to light on a coat sleeve, white stars melting even as they strike. How did such force and beauty come to be in something so small and fleeting and unknowable? You did not have to understand miracles to believe in them, and in fact Mabel had come to suspect the opposite. To believe, perhaps you had to cease looking for explanations and instead hold the little thing in your hands as long as you were able before it slipped like water between your fingers."

The tale follows the couple's growth and reconnection as they rediscover the beauty of the world surrounding them, illuminating a powerful and stirring message of the power of mindfulness and faith. In the beginning of the story, Mabel is preoccupied by the past and by the loss of her child; her healing begins once she becomes aware of the intoxicating landscape that surrounds her—and of the appearance of a lovely fairy-like child who appears from the woods, apparently sculpted out of snow, and who disappears and reappears like memories do.

> "Begin at once to live, and count each separate
> day as a separate life." –Seneca

NOW

Mabel fights and ultimately overcomes her grief by practicing mindfulness, albeit inadvertently, and by training her brain to see, hear, and sense everyday miracles. Her path towards healing and fulfillment parallels the points of the NOW acronym...

✧ Notice.

As Mabel begins to notice the beauty of her surroundings in the present moment, she actively opens her mind to perceive the miracles of nature and life.

✧ Opportunities.

Mabel seized an opportunity to strengthen her character and heal her heart by opening her mind to the possibilities of the present moment, choosing consciously not to dwell on the past or to be tormented by the uncertainty of the future.

✦ Within.

In doing so, Mabel was able to go within herself to see how her past tragedy prevented life in the present.

> "Reflect upon your present blessings, of which every man has plenty; not on your past misfortunes, of which all men have some." –Charles Dickens

THE PATH TO MINDFULNESS

Your brain is what constructs your reality, based on the input from your senses. Sound waves and light waves, for instance, are converted into inner images and processed as experiences. If you are preoccupied by inner images from the past or the future, you miss the sentient present. Although you think that your brain is providing you with a vision of an objective reality, nothing could be further from the truth. Neuroscientists have shown that we mold and decipher what we see according to our personal preconceived notions.

The good news? The brain constantly rewires itself—so you have the power to reframe and reshape your reality.

Through the practice of mindfulness, we can train our brains to consciously filter in everyday miracles through our senses—such as the sight of blooming flowers, the fragrance of the ocean, or the caress of the wind. The deliberate focus on the present moment through your senses signals to your brain that it can feel safe and grounded—and this in turn helps it secrete "happiness chemicals" like dopamine and endorphins.

PRACTICE

One of the easiest and most effective ways to reconnect with life is simply to take a stroll through nature. But not just any sort of stroll. Not a preoccupied, walking-but-not-really-seeing-ahead-of-me stroll. A mindful stroll. A conscious, 100%-in-the-moment stroll.

Spend some time each day enjoying a mindful walk. Let your attention drop into your senses and absorb the abundance of sensations bombarding you. As you walk, notice what you see, hear, feel, and even taste. Instead of focusing on your racing or interrupting thoughts, deliberately choose to notice your present surroundings. Gently return to the details of the *now*. Raindrops... sunlight... flowers, leaves, snowflakes... the feel of the ground beneath your feet... the sensation of your arms swinging as you walk... the feeling of the fresh air against your face.

These are the little things in life, which are truly the magnificent and big things. You will find that the more grateful you are, the more you will have to be grateful for. Open up your mind to the life around you. Take time to inwardly express gratitude for the miracles of nature. By practicing this faithfully, you will master the art of attuning your senses to pay attention to the present.

"We never know what is going to happen,
do we? Life is always throwing us this way
and that. That's where the adventure is. Not
knowing where you'll end up or how you'll fare.
It's all a mystery, and when we say any different,
we're just lying to ourselves. Tell me, when have
you felt most alive?" *–The Snow Child*

THE MINDFULNESS
MENTALITY

A PIECE OF MIND FOR YOUR PEACE OF MIND: LIVING WITH MINDFULNESS

☑ *Can you recall the last time that you heard the warbling birds piercing the sky with their vibrant notes of song? You've heard it, but you've made birdsong a background noise; when did you last consciously listen?*

☑ *Did you see and acknowledge the kind smile of the person who held the elevator for you, or who opened the door for you, or who stopped their car for you so that you could safely cross the road in front of them?*

☑ *When your loved ones, friends, or coworkers excitedly relate their accomplishments or experiences, how do you react? Do you genuinely share in their happiness? Do you allow their contagious emotions to affect you?*

☑ *When someone speaks to you, do you actively listen? Do you fully engage in conversations with family members? Do you let yourself live in the moment?*

THE POWER OF FELICITY

The words "consciously", "allow", and "let" are not coincidental in the above questions.

All too often, we are so caught up in the everyday tempest of activity and routine, that we lose sight of our purpose. We lose sight of the meaning we've assigned to life. We forget that each day could be our last day—for if we knew this, and we had a choice, surely we'd spend the "last day" differently. We forget to live and so we merely survive, going through the motions.

There is nothing sadder than this throwing away of our liberty to live life to the fullest. But as sad as it is, it's just as easy to reconnect with our innermost selves and realign our lives with purpose and joy—as long as we decide that we *want* to.

In his book *A Simple Heart,* French novelist Gustave Flaubert examines the life of a maid named Felicite (a word that literally means "intense happiness"), who would appear to have an insignificant job and humdrum life. Flaubert wrote the book during an era when servitude was popular; he crafted Felicite as an extremely poor young woman who endured great hardships before being employed by a well-to-do family. Flaubert breaks through biases and assumptions to delve into Felicite's mind and reveal to his readers a rich inner world that, initially, may seem oxymoronic or ironic given Felicite's situation and lifestyle. She is described as a kind-hearted and loving soul, with deep gratitude for the little and simple things in life. Everyday situations rouse her soul and cause her to display traits of tenderness and a deep reverence for life.

Flaubert basically illuminates the concept that we make our own sunshine; that happiness is an inside job; that a place doesn't make a person—it is the person who makes a place.

NOW

The Felicites of the world are invaluable individuals—and they have much to teach us. They have found the key to happiness—that "secret" that so many books and movies and schools of thought chase—and they've unlocked the door that leads to their better selves. They live by the "NOW" Principle...

❖ Notice.

To notice, in this context, means *to be aware*. But it's about empathy as much as is it about attention and focus. Felicite had the willingness to put herself in other people's shoes, to share in their triumphs and tribulations, and to emotionally become attune to their feelings and experiences.

❖ Opportunities.

Felicite created opportunities to feel deep connection and compassion. There is a scene where she experiences the first Communion of a child named Virginie, who is under Felicite's care. Felicite imagines herself in Virginie's shoes, receiving Communion, and she shares in the child's experience of profound wonder and spirituality.

❖ Within.

Though Felicite's life may have seemed, to an impartial outsider, like a shabby canvas of poverty and drudgery, her inner world was anything but! It was rich and vibrant; she lived life to the fullest, and thus her life was fulfilling.

This is done through mindfulness.

"If you want to be happy, be." -Leo Tolstoy

THE PATH TO MINDFULNESS

As a psychotherapist, I've had the opportunity and privilege to experience stories of people from all walks of life. When I used to perform psychological testing for a back rehabilitation program, I had the pleasure of meeting a man with Felicite's mindset. He suffered from a severe back injury due to many years of physical labor. Yet his inner world was pure and his disposition shed sunrays wherever he went. Like Felicite, he was extremely low-profile and easily overlooked, yet his inner world was very rich and filled with appreciation for the experience of the present moment.

I've noted the opposite scenario with many clients. Many of them come with questions about why they feel unhappy despite external and material success. I remind them that happiness is an inside job. It is not composed of tangible things. It is not even composed of exterior things. Happiness springs from our inner world. Once they realize this—that they can find happiness by creating it themselves—my clients can begin to unleash their newfound power: the ability to create inner joy. This book is based on literary examples of people who have transcended harsh circumstances and found inner peace…. they serve as exemplars and inspiration.

What is mindfulness, exactly? How does it work? Mindfulness enables us to accept *what is*, and reminds us of *how to live and love with passion and compassion*. It is the ability to embrace the present, to experience and express gratitude, and to delve deep into the heart of an issue.

You begin by paying attention to your inner life. How do you feel? What are you thinking about? You are able to condition and alter your behavior and your mindset, but first you must define it. Begin to notice the voices in your head, objectively, as you would eavesdrop on a conversation—do you speak kindly or harshly to yourself? Note your thoughts, without judgement. See them as words written on the whiteboard of your mind, then visualize yourself picking up an eraser and wiping them away. Imagine a clean board, and then fill it with kinder words instead.

PRACTICE

Take five minutes each day. Just sit quietly and notice your thoughts. Let them flit freely through your mind. You'll notice how your thoughts and reactions have been conditioned. You'll notice what triggers them. You'll notice how your body reacts—like when it becomes tense or your breathing quickens after a negative train of thought.

The purpose of this practice isn't to make you a passive observer. You are just taking in the information, first. Once you see what triggers things, you'll be able to step in and change them. Seize each opportunity to do so. You can hit pause, rewind, and remake the movie in your mind. And, with enough practice, you'll be able to play the movie positively the first time around. Guide yourself so that your thoughts become constructive, rather than destructive. Nurture your soul and wellbeing by practicing gratitude. Instead of looking at what's going wrong... turn your mind's eye—at least for a moment, *right now*—and focus on what's going right.

→ What are you grateful for in the present moment? Your health, your surroundings, your family?

→ What blessings can you notice that you ordinarily take for granted?

→ How can you live today as if it is your only day?

"Most folks are about as happy as they make up their minds to be." –Abraham Lincoln

FREEDOM WITHIN: HOW MINDFULNESS LIBERATED ANNE FRANK

☑ *Are you often overwhelmed by dread or uncertainty regarding the future?*

☑ *Do you feel helpless, as if someone else is writing the story of your life?*

☑ *Are you troubled by self-pity?*

WARRIOR OF PEACE

Her diary became the most popular journal in the history of literature. Her optimism, strength of will, and outlook became a beacon of inspiration for millions of readers. Her writing became her legacy, a ray of sunshine shining out from one of the darkest eras of human history...

Her name was Anne Frank, and she was only thirteen years old when she began writing in her diary during the German occupation of Amsterdam during WWII, in the midst of the Holocaust. For two years, she secretly wrote in her diary, hidden in the secret annex of a crumbling warehouse with her family—until 1944, when her family was discovered and sent to die in concentration camps. Only her father survived; he published Anne's diary a few years later.

Despite the horrific setting, the unthinkable terrors unfolding around her, and the impending permanent doom of potentially being betrayed, discovered, and killed, Anne's diary mirrors an outlook that is remarkably positive, courageous, and pure. She knew, true to her words, that "whoever is happy will make others happy too." She'd discovered the power and peace that comes from cultivating a rich inner world, and she made a choice—knowing that time was limited—to live each day as if it were her last, because the odds said that it could be.

"Everyone has inside of him a piece of good news. The good news is that you don't know how great you can be! How much you can love! What you can accomplish! And what your potential is!" –Anne Frank: The Diary of a Young Girl

NOW

In order to survive, Anne had to find an outlet for expression, for venting, for creativity, and for a way to pass the time. She chose to keep a diary. It was the most important thing she'd ever done.

✧ Notice.

Writing down her thoughts enabled Anne to consciously notice, dissect, and explore them as she chronicled them.

✧ Opportunities.

Her diary encouraged her to live each moment and make it as memorable as possible, something worth writing and philosophizing about. It gave her an opportunity to feel like the protagonist and scriptwriter of her own life, despite all the conditions and catalysts that fought against that freedom. It gave her a chance to unleash her feelings, her thoughts, her fears, and her joys.

✧ Within.

It helped her explore her inner world and her outlook on the events within the annex and in the tumultuous world beyond. It helped ground her in her moments of fear, pain, and doubt, and soothed her by reminding her of all she'd experienced, of her accomplishments, of her dreams, and of her aspirations.

"How wonderful it is that nobody need wait a single moment before starting to improve the world." –Anne Frank

THE PATH TO MINDFULNESS

As I write this post, I am in a doctor's waiting room, waiting to be called into his office. I am undergoing a consultation for a surgery. Remembering Anne Frank reminds me to focus on the gifts of the present moment. Even in a stressful situation, I realize that we always have opportunities to practice mindfulness. Her words remind me of the "freedom in ourselves" to choose our own thoughts and outlook. And so I decide to do just that.

I notice the bright colors of the room and the soothing whir of the air conditioner. Focusing my attention on positive, cheery sights and sounds does not change the reality—the fact that I must face a necessary surgery—but it does help me feel calmer and more centered. Why waste this opportunity to focus on the present moment? My medical problems remind me that our health and life circumstance can change abruptly and without warning—which is all the more reason to cherish whatever we have, when we have it. I deliberately focus my attention on the bright blue of my shirt and the crisp white of my pants... breathing, noticing, breathing, noticing...

"Never let the future disturb you. You will meet it, if you have to, with all the same weapons of reason which today arm you against the present." –Marcus Aurelius

PRACTICE

When you find yourself in a challenging situation that leaves you feeling tense or quaking, the best and quickest thing you can do is simply breathe—deeply, purposefully, and deliberately slow. Think "BE" each time you inhale... think "CALM" each time you exhale.

As you feel yourself calming down—because your body will immediately and literally feel the tension melting out of you as your steady breathing begins to regulate the behavior and flow of energy through your body—continue this exercise deliberately and repetitively. Keep your eyes closed. After a few moments, open your eyes and intentionally notice your surroundings. See the sights and colors around you. Note the sounds. Feel your own weight against the surface you are sitting or lying on. Feel what sensations are against your hands and feet. Center your body in the present moment.

As I practice this breathing technique here in the waiting room of the doctor's office, waiting for my doctor to present to me the surgery options, I notice that the wallpaper is a lovely beige-and-blue pattern with pleasant muted pyramids. There is a small cloisonné mirror in a corner that I've never noticed before. I hear the strains of a familiar song that transport me to a happier time.

The act of reminding ourselves that "all there is is the now"—and focusing on the gifts of the present moment—is calming and particularly auspicious when we find ourselves in stressful circumstances.

"Think of all the beauty still left around you
and be happy." –Anne Frank

THE SENSATION OF
LIVING IN THE NOW

☑ *Do you frequently stress about yesterday and worry about tomorrow?*

☑ *Are you afraid that you'll run out of time or that you're somehow missing out on life?*

☑ *Do you ever stop to register how your entire body is feeling?*

☑ *When was the last time you were consciously grateful to be alive?*

FEARFULLY AND WONDERFULLY MADE

"I have sometimes wondered why Jesus so frequently touched the people he healed, many of whom must have been unattractive, obviously diseased, unsanitary, smelly... He could have divided the crowd into affinity groups and organized his miracles--paralyzed people over there, feverish people here, people with leprosy there--raising his hands to heal each group efficiently, en masse. But he chose not to. [...] He wanted those people, one by one, to feel his love and warmth and his full identification with them. Jesus knew he could not readily demonstrate love to a crowd, for love usually involves touching."

The above quote is derived from the inspirational book *Fearfully and Wonderfully Made*, written by Philip Yancy and surgeon Dr. Paul Brand.

Included in the book are Dr. Brand's reflections about his time spent with people suffering from leprosy, revealing how that experience altered his life by making him appreciate the function of the human skin and its ability to feel sensations. Leprosy is a condition that causes granulomas of the nerves, respiratory tract, eyes, and skin; it results in a person's inability to feel. Apart from the skin lesions and damage due to the disease itself, lepers are typically covered with sores that are caused when they sit on something hard or when they lean on sharp objects. Wounds and infections can result in tissue loss and deformation, numbed and diseased skin, and permanent damage to the nerves, limbs, and eyes.

We often take the gift of our five senses for granted. Yet just stop a moment and imagine having no feeling in your skin to warn you of extreme heat, sharp objects, or dangerous situations. Dr. Brand imagined this frequently. Although leprosy can be treated, it is contagious via nasal droplets; the doctor often wondered if he would wake up with the numbing symptoms. It changed his outlook and made him intensely grateful for the sensation of touch that we take for granted.

> "Live each day like it's your last, because someday you're going to be right." –Mohammad Ali

NOW

Live the day like it's your last. Take a moment and just look around you, see what draws your attention and what pleases your eyes. Allow your attention to focus on that someone or something for 30 seconds. Of course other thoughts will enter your mind meanwhile. Notice them, acknowledge them, but don't let them distract you from your object. You may notice a greater sense of relaxation and calm as you immerse yourself in the experience of the present moment.

✧ Notice... what your body is showing you.

✧ Opportunities... to be conscious and grateful are plentiful.

✧ Within... the path to conscious feeling and thinking and healing begins from stimuli like touch but resonates within you.

"There is only one time that is important: now! It is the most important time because it is the only time when we have any power." –Leo Tolstoy

THE PATH TO MINDFULNESS

Pema Chodron is among those who take mindfulness one step further. She is an American-born Tibetan Buddhist, ordained nun, and author. She strongly advocates the Buddhist meditation practice called *Tonglen*, which is Tibetan for "sending and receiving". This technique is about visualizing *taking in* suffering—one's personal suffering and/or the suffering of others—with each inhaling breath, and *giving out* acknowledgment, compassion, solidarity, and aid during each exhaling breath. In this practice, you make room in your heart and mind for suffering and breathe out healing to yourself and others who are experiencing similar pain. Breathe in pain, fear, or anger; breathe out healing for yourself and others who are stuck in similar states of suffering.

Literally illogical, perhaps, but psychologically powerful. This technique has been shown to cultivate mind patterns which promote an attitude of love and self-sacrifice, where you can exchange pain for love and happiness. In practice, it can increase your own peace of mind, thereby spreading more harmony and happiness to your surroundings. Dr. Brand felt compassion and identification with the patients that helped transform his inner life and bring healing to others.

Personally I have had the privilege of working with a group of terminally ill cancer patients. What floored me was their vibrancy, their joie de vivre; they took such delight in every moment because they knew that their lives would soon end. Mindfulness is about the celebration of the miracle of life that we so often take for granted. Everyday miracles, "simple" miracles, such as seeing, feeling, hearing, smelling, and tasting—these are so overlooked, so underrated, yet so important. If we thought that we were going to wake up tomorrow and not be able to see, feel, smell, or hear, then we would cherish our senses more.

PRACTICE

If you've never tried this before—of if you're looking for a different method to practice mindfulness more effectively—the "body scan" is an excellent technique to get in touch with your senses on a daily basis and monitor how you're doing and feeling...

→ Sit or lie down, and take three deep breaths. Mentally count each inhalation/exhalation.

→ Focus on your body for a few moments. Notice where you feel tension, pressure, or tightness. Simply allow your attention to scan through your body, as if you're taking an X-ray. Become aware of all the sensations.

→ Remind yourself that the intention of this practice is to focus on bodily sensations and to notice what happens. Watch without judgment. Observe the sensations of the present moment.

→ Let yourself be curious about the sensations in your body and the places where you've been unconsciously tense and pressured all this time. How strong are the sensations? How tight is the pressure? Is there throbbing? What parts of your body are in need of attention and healing? Remember—it is essential to be kind and objective during your self-diagnosis.

→ Re-scan your body more selectively and thoroughly. Begin with your head. Notice any pressure or tension. Drop your awareness to your neck and shoulders. Then your chest—often a place where a lot of tension brews. Next let your focus shift to your abdomen, your belly, and your back. Shift your attention down to your legs, moving further down till you reach the soles of your feet and the tips of your toes.

→ Meanwhile, stretch each muscle as you go—and, as you visualize the knots loosening, imagine that this is due to the healing energy you are sending through your body. Repeat the mantra of loving kindness mentally or out loud: *May I be healed. May I be at peace. May I be filled with loving kindness.*

→ Repeat as needed throughout the day. Cherish your body and send oxygen, intentional healing, and loving compassion to all the areas that need to relax.

Remember that there is no one right way to do this. You'll do what feels right for you. The purpose of this exercise is simply to divert your attention into your body and to observe inner sensations with curiosity, openness, and gratitude. Just remember to stay centered and focused on the feelings and sensations. You can do body scans many times throughout the day, reminding your body that you don't need to hold onto negative thoughts or toxic emotions. You can mindfully and gently release tension and start afresh.

"Although time seems to fly by, it never travels faster than one day at a time. Each day is a new opportunity to live your life to the fullest." –Steve Maraboli

MINDFULNESS AS THE ROAD TO RECOVERY

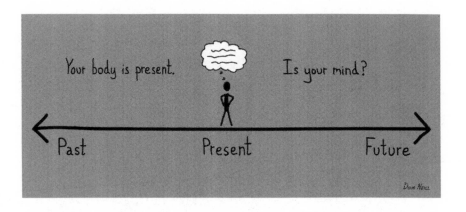

THE ART OF MENTAL REWRITING: REFRAMING MEMORIES TO REVAMP PERSPECTIVES

☑ *Do you find that your present experiences trigger toxic past memories?*

☑ *Are you plagued by negative experiences that deprive you of joy and self-love?*

☑ *Do you often blow things out of proportion, or find it difficult to let go of negativity?*

MENTAL TRIGGERS

French novelist, essayist, and critic Marcel Proust left a legacy of thought and philosophy. In his writing, he explores themes of memory and identity. One of his most pronounced motifs—that we have the ability to reconstruct our mental vision of the past in our minds—is a cornerstone of mindfulness. In the text below—an excerpt from *Volume 1: Swann's Way*[1]

---

[1] The definitive French Pleiade edition translated by C.K. Scott Moncrieff and Terence Kilmartin. New York: Vintage. pp. 48-51.

---

of his seven-volume novel *Remembrance of Things Past*[2]—Proust describes the memories triggered by biting into a cookie:

"...As soon as I had recognized the taste of the piece of madeleine soaked in her decoction of lime-blossom which my aunt used to give me (although I didn't not yet know and must long postpone the discovery of why this memory made me so happy) immediately the old grey house upon the street, where her room was, rose up like a stage set to attach itself to the little pavilion opening on to the garden which had been built out behind it for my parents (the isolated segment which until that moment had been all that I could see): and with it the house of the town, from morning to night and in all the weathers, the Square where I used to be sent before lunch, the streets along which I used to run errands, the country roads we took when it was fine."

Proust describes a completely natural phenomenon. Since memories can be instantly evoked by any of the five senses—the fragrance of a mother's perfume, the taste of fried bacon, the vision of an angry parent's scowl, the sound of frozen tree branches breaking under the weight of ice, the texture of a velvet dress against our skin—it's easy to imagine how many till-then-forgotten memories the mere taste of a familiar cookie might trigger.

> "Happiness depends more on the inward disposition of mind than on outward circumstances." –Benjamin Franklin

NOW

Practicing mindfulness—being focused and aware of your subjective consciousness from a first-person perspective—will enable you to use the NOW approach, a process which helps you become aware of associations so that you can promote positivity and dismiss negativity.

---

[2]   Also translated as *In Search of Lost Time.*

✧ Notice.

The first step is to become aware of how your body responds to triggers, especially in ways that no longer serve you. For instance, you may realize that you tense up and start stressing out every time your boss scowls.

✧ Opportunities.

Once you realize the reaction, you can then see the strength of this physical and emotional response. Your brain creates stories to protect you, so there's always a reasoning—an old story—behind a specific feeling. Step back and question if your feelings are prejudiced by past experiences or the present situation.

✧ Within.

Once you define what's going on, you can consciously decide to deal with it, and to develop different habits. When did you first learn this feeling, this fear? Examine the story origins: perhaps you once had a parent who scowled to intimidate you before punishing you. You've stored that fear subconsciously, and it resurfaces—in all its numbing intensity—when you see someone scowl. Ask if that protective old story still serves you. Does it make you better or bitter?

Once you decide to make a change, you're on the right track... but your journey isn't over yet. You've reminded yourself that you can rewrite the story. And now that's exactly what you must do.

> "Nothing can stop the person with the right
> mental attitude from achieving his goal.
> Nothing on earth can help the person with the
> wrong attitude." –Thomas Jefferson

THE PATH TO MINDFULNESS

An evoked memory, of course, may be positive or negative. Whether it is one or the other is based on two things: your past experience when you actually lived through and created that memory, and—since then—your mental association with that memory. Positive memories contribute to our wellbeing and happiness, melding to create a springboard that encourages us to love life and confidently tackle new adventures. Negative experiences are a part of life, too; good decisions come from experience, and experience comes from bad decisions. However, it's just as essential to learn lessons and then let things go. When blown out of proportion or when we refuse to let them go, negative memories can deprive us of our joie de vivre, our confidence, and our self-love. Our brain stores all of these memories and they can be evoked in an instant—we may not even be aware that our mood has shifted.

And yet they have the power to ultimately destroy us.

So how do we counter them? Each one of us has the power to transform the negative into positive—we need only harness this power. *You* must pick up the pen and write the story of your life… or someone else will. Reframe your memories. Rewrite your stories. By changing your story, you change your life.

PRACTICE

Think of the story of your memory like a drawing. A bunch of scribbles, say. How will you frame it? If a five-year-old came up to you and handed you those scribbles, you'd smile and congratulate the child… but the drawing would probably wind up in the trash (when the kid wasn't looking, of course!). But if you saw that same scribbled drawing beautifully framed and hoisted on an art gallery wall, because it was drawn by some incredible minimalist artist whose name you can't really pronounce, then the *same exact drawing* might be suddenly worth millions of dollars!

It's the same drawing… it's just that the context has changed!

You can choose to focus on a positive aspect of that memory, to spin it in your favor. This is a deliberate choice. And you can find ways to help your "rewrite" sink in, too—the tapping technique, for instance. Motion causes emotion, but it's also about the power of association, so think of it as a way to amplify the rewritten memory: gently tap bilaterally on each knee for a total of six taps as you recall a time when you felt peaceful and happy. Maybe it's a memory of you at the beach... on a mountain trip... curled up with your loved one... or whatever other memory can't help but make you smile.

Why? Because in the brain, practice makes permanence. Over time, your mind will associate this particular pattern of tapping with that particular feel-good memory. At times when you're under stress, you can use this bilateral tapping technique as a reminder to visit your "happy place" and immediately alleviate the stress by countering a negative experience with a happy memory.

> "If a problem can't be solved within the frame it was conceived, the solution lies in reframing the problem." –Brian McGreevy

MENTAL SUICIDE: THE DANGER OF GRUDGES AND HOW TO LET GO

☑ *Do you struggle to forgive yourself or others?*

☑ *Are you overwhelmed by anger, bitterness, or toxic emotions?*

☑ *Do you feel unable to think positively about a person or a situation which you consider unforgivable?*

☑ *Are there many things you consider unforgivable?*

TO SPARE A MOCKINGBIRD

In Harper Lee's internationally acclaimed novel, *To Kill a Mockingbird*, the author transports us to the heart of the American South during the 1930s. Lee introduces us to her female protagonist, an adventurous girl named Scout. There's a scene where Scout is fighting other children because they are ridiculing her father, Atticus Finch. Atticus is a soft-spoken, whip-smart attorney who has shouldered a difficult case, defending a black man in court. Atticus isn't proud of his daughter's brawl, and advises her accordingly: "You just hold your head up high and keep those fists down...

No matter what anybody says to you, don't let 'em get your goat. Try fighting with your head for a change."

Atticus is basically preaching two things—forgiveness, a medicine that is even more potent for the forgiver than the forgiven; and clear-headed logic, which enables us to step back and see the big picture, to assess the intensity and importance of a situation, to pick our battles, and to let go of that which has no right to weigh us down.

> "Forgiveness does not change the past, but it does enlarge the future." –Paul Boese

NOW

In his way, Atticus encourages mindfulness. Without practicing conscious thought, we don't realize how our subconscious brain actually stores maladaptive experiences—purely with good intentions, since our brain seeks to protect us, and lashes out with defensive thoughts against others or even ourselves. In essence, though, these backstories backfire; "the hysterical is historical" you could say, because a reaction that is much stronger than the infraction is a reaction that emerges from past conditioning.

✧ Notice...

For instance, if you're sitting in a staff meeting and can't stop mentally attacking a coworker whom you hardly know, it helps to remind yourself that this is NOW. Examine why your reaction is so strong. Often it is because you are reminded of a maladaptive pattern or person from your past (and this may have absolutely nothing to do with the present situation).

✧ Opportunities...

When you bring those thoughts into the light of consciousness, you have a choice of what to think. You have an opportunity to change. You can decide to stop the attacking thoughts which are generating an overdose of adrenaline and cortisol, making you tense and unhappy.

✧ Within…

You know how awful it feels after you get riled up, after the heat of your unchecked anger simmers down to become a cold lump of resentment. You know how awful it feels to direct toxic thoughts against someone else—you are projecting your grudge, even if you don't speak. If you just stop to think about it, holding on to anger and bitterness doesn't hurt anyone else more than it hurts you. The negativity and anger brims and simmers within *you*, destroying *you*. Holding on to anger is like drinking poison and expecting someone else to die.

"Lord, grant me the strength to accept the things I cannot change, the courage to change the things I can, and the wisdom to know the difference." –Francis of Assisi

THE PATH OF MINDFULNESS

Mindfulness helps children like Scout hold their head up high, their fists down, and to keep others away from "getting their goat". They learn to use their head to handle disputes. *The Journal for Family* (2013) reported that in a study of 400 children, mindfulness training resulted in significant increases in the students' attention, self-control, classroom participation, and respect for others. Consequently, there's been further interest in using mindfulness as an educational tactic. The UCLA Mindfulness Awareness Research Center found improvements in the self-regulatory abilities of preschoolers and elementary school students after they participated in just eight weeks of mindfulness training—and children who initially were most challenged by self-regulation showed the strongest improvements.

Although it is ideal to begin this practice at a young age, it is never too late to begin to strengthen your inborn capability to self-regulate. Your brain retains its plasticity for a lifetime; you need never stop growing and learning. It is never too late to heed the advice of Atticus Finch by refusing to allow others to "get your goat".

The mindful practice of noticing our thoughts is what increases our awareness of how we react based on past hurts and resentments. It decreases our stress levels, enables us to think more clearly, to consider the consequences, and to fathom and accept someone else's point of view. Forgiveness is the next step—the release of those hurts and resentments, and the catharsis that ensues from this.

"Forgiving isn't something you do for someone else. It's something you do for yourself. It's saying, *You're not important enough to have a stranglehold on me.* It's saying, *You don't get to trap me in the past. I am worthy of a future.*" –Jodi Picoult, *The Storyteller*

PRACTICE

Practice this next time you find yourself in such a situation. Visualize your muscles as knots. Drop your attention into your body and assess how you are holding your muscles. You're probably extremely tense. Your body might, in fact, even be physically hurting or uncomfortable from the amount of pressure you're putting on it. Imagine that you find these knots and you are loosening them. You are letting go of stress.

Instead of *reacting*, try *responding*. Shift your awareness to the attacking thoughts and focus on a compassionate mantra, a kindness meditation:

May I be healed. May I be at peace. May I be filled with loving kindness.

Like Scout, there are many people who are plagued by anger, a sense of injustice and bitterness, and negativity. Of course you must stand up for what is right, of course you should act upon your honor and integrity, and of course you are not supposed to swallow all the wrongs of the world. But, like Atticus, you must know that there is a better way. This way is more peaceful yet more effective in the long-term. The way of non-violence, of calm reassessment, of logic and love powerful enough to be reckoned with. The way that keeps your blood level and heart rate and stress chemicals in check, and keeps you happy and alive for longer.

TRIGGER-HAPPY: HOW TO REWIRE "RELIVING" AND PRACTICE "REWRITING"

☑ *Do you find yourself struggling to feel heard, seen, or understood in your relationships?*

☑ *Do you lash out against others or against yourself over the "little things", and have you ever wondered if this is symbolic of an underlying issue that you are not addressing?*

☑ *Do you often submit to "worst case scenario" thought patterns?*

TRIGGERS AND FLASHBACKS

Cultural identity and complexity, human empathy, and control over one's personal destiny—these are all themes enmeshed in the writings of Amy Tan, Californian-born Chinese-American author. In one of her acclaimed books—*The Opposite of Fate: Memories of a Writing Life*—Amy Tan illuminates how the brain can be instantaneously triggered by current events to flash back to past stories, and how challenging it can be to gain equilibrium in the present moment. She also examines how personal ideologies frame our own realities, including the world of memory we contain in our minds: *"Isn't the past what people remember—who did what, how and why? And what the people remember, isn't that mostly what they've already chosen to believe?"*

These themes translate into Amy Tan's everyday personal life as much as they do in her writings. She says that she avoids reading reviews of her books in order to avoid "[putting] a symbolic cream pie in the face of negative reviewers". But she can't escape them altogether; occasionally, she says, a well-meaning friend will bring a negative review to her attention. It is difficult for her to see the bright side of such criticism, even as she knows that her defensiveness stems from a very deep-rooted pain from past traumas: "It is dreadful to hear things like that and I am reduced to the emotional level of a six-year-old outcast taunted at school for bringing Chinese food in her lunch bag," she admits. "The words remain as indelible as cat piss on my bed pillow."

"Neurons that fire together wire together." –Donald Hebb

NOW

When we shift from reliving past traumas to actively countering the triggers with mindful compassion, we begin to rewire our brains, paving the way to a more beneficial direction. Even a few daily moments of mindfulness can retrain the nervous system to secrete wellness-promoting chemicals and revel in the positive aspects of our relationships. With practice, of course, the brain becomes even more efficient at accomplishing this. The steps of the NOW approach can help us break down the process...

❖ Notice.

Amy Tan was able to notice when she was reliving past childhood distress. By acknowledging her issues, she was able to consciously face them and analyze ways to deter and overcome them.

❖ Opportunities.

Amy Tan then realized that she had a choice to accept or block the negative mental repercussions of those triggers. She could choose what she listened to, what feedback she accepted, and how she allowed the feedback to affect her.

✧ Within.

Amy Tan shows how, by delving into herself and focusing on the blessings of her life as a successful author and loving wife, she can remind and rewire her brain to differentiate between the *then* and the *now*. By going within, she gave words to her experiences, and literally turned them into a story that helped her detach and even find humor in the image of a symbolic cream pie.

"There is one thing we always need, and that is the watchman named Mindfulness—the guard who is always on the lookout for when we get carried away by Mindlessness." –Tulku Urgyen

THE PATH TO MINDFULNESS

Amy Tan's experience—of the brain dropping back into old memories and associations, triggered by current events that remind us of past experiences—is what psychotherapists call "reliving". It happens to all of us; it's the experience of dropping into the mental "black hole", so to speak. This can be particularly obvious when examining relationships; we can say or do things that advertently or inadvertently trigger a memory of past hurt in our partner's mind, causing that person to return to that hurtful past experience and become upset and unreasonable. That person acts out due to the past pain; the ensuing chaos is called a "train wreck".

I recently saw a client—let's call her Pamela—who, though now an adult, is still traumatized by the bullying she endured as a child decades ago; she'd been taunted—as Amy Tan had been—because she was ethnically different from the others. So many years later, this pain would emerge during arguments with her partner, Mike. Whenever Pamela discerned criticism in Mike's voice, she overreacted and withdrew into stony silence. This in turn would trigger Mike's own insecurities and pain; Pamela's silence made Mike feel abandoned, an emotion compounded by his past (in which his father left his family and his mother spiraled into depression). Pamela and Mike thus developed a destructive "train wreck" pattern.

These train wrecks can be formidable forces, even destroying relationships. With the practice of mindful compassion, however, they can be countered. When both partners work to practice mindful compassion instead of merely emotionally reacting, they can change the dynamic between them. They become better, not bitter.

There is nothing more human than our intrinsic need to feel loved and appreciated. Our brains are literally wired for connection; we evolved together in groups, after all. Relationship researchers actually have a term for our deep fear of losing important social connections: *attachment panic*. Mindfulness helps us become aware of this fear and enables us to compassionately face it instead of negatively acting out. We can thus avoid train wrecks while helping one another heal from past distresses.

As a therapist, I've noticed that when couples become more compassionate towards one another—by being more empathetic, understanding the past pain of their partner—they feel better. Psychologist and author Harville Hendrix has termed it this way: "We never do something to our partner that we are not also doing to ourselves." The benefits of our happiness manifest physically as well as mentally: compassion releases feel-good chemicals like oxytocin and dopamine, quashing negative triggered chemicals such as adrenalin and cortisol.

PRACTICE

Neuropsychologist Rick Hanson suggests the practice of following a negative memory with a positive memory. It's about practicing mindful awareness that you are "reliving" things during an experience or a conflict, and you choose to deliberately instill some positivity. In the situation of Pamela and Mike, for instance, here is how that would play out:

→ **Awareness**: Pamela, lashing out at Mike's "criticism" in self-righteous and defensive anger, would become aware of her defensiveness and overreaction.

→ **Analysis:** Pamela would remind herself that she was reliving old feelings of hurt and anger that she'd felt when being bullied by other children for being different.

→ **Notice:** She would then notice how she was taking her pain out on Mike, backfiring her past onto him. Mike would also notice the ways in which his past threatened to supersede his love for and connection to his wife.

→ **Mindfulness:** Both partners would need to practice mindful listening. When one person spoke, the other one wouldn't interrupt and would pay close attention. Both would notice when their thoughts began to wander off or when emotion started overcoming their thought patterns. They would catch themselves "reliving"; each time, they would practice transitioning from "reliving" to "rewiring" through reconnecting and actively listening.

→ **Response:** Each partner would work on *responding* in a compassionate way—instead of *reacting*. This would help to fuel their relationship with emotions of love rather than fear.

> "Some researchers have proposed that experiencing empathy and compassion through the mirror neuron system is equivalent to having compassion for yourself. Thus, 'giving is receiving' is a brain-based truth. Insensitivity and selfishness are essentially bad for your brain and your mental health. In contrast, compassion and loving relationships are good for your brain and your mental health." –John B. Arden, *Rewire Your Brain: Think Your Way to a Better Life*

MINDFULNESS AS A PATH OF SELF-DISCOVERY

OUT OF YOUR HEAD
AND INTO YOUR SOUL

☑ *Do you fear that you're missing out on life?*

☑ *Are you waiting for something? To be loved? To be successful? To be happy?*

☑ *Do you often feel like life is simply carrying you along, as something beyond your control?*

THE NARCISSIST

In ancient Greek mythology, Narcissus was a beautiful youth who caught sight of his reflection in a pond one day and became completely enamored with it. It is said that he lay down by the water to gaze at his face, growing obsessed with his own image. Since he was unable to obtain the object of his desire, he died where he lay, overcome by grief. Sounds pathetic, but in many instances it's a frighteningly accurate metaphor. The term "narcissist" is derived from this myth, and it tellingly refers to a person who is self-enamored and self-preoccupied, often to an obsessive and dangerous degree.

In his novella *The Beast in the Jungle,* author Henry James introduces us to exactly such a character: John Marcher, an extremely self-centered young man who is convinced that he has been selected by fate for a special event that will occur in his lifetime. He encounters a sensitive and intelligent young woman, May Bartram, who listens to John's theory concerning his personal foreboding and conviction that he's destined for greatness. May offers her friendship and agrees to watch and wait with John until this special fate comes to fruition. For many years, John sits idly and refuses to let May get close to him, ignoring the love of a good woman and killing time as he waits for his "spectacular fate".

The story unravels to become a tale of lost life and lost love; it is only after May dies that John realizes that he's missed most of his life—and the opportunity for true love—while waiting for a rare, strange, and self-concocted "event" that never happens. By living in his head and focusing on a fantasy, he missed the true meaning of life. He missed out on friendship, love, purpose, adventure, discovery, and self-growth. Gambling for nothing, he lost everything.

> "In this moment, there is plenty of time.
> In this moment, you are precisely as you
> should be. In this moment, there is infinite
> possibility." –Victoria Moran

NOW

As mindfulness is all about "living in the now", the idea suitably circles back to the NOW philosophy...

✧ Notice.

Look around you and experience the life and love that surrounds you. It is right beside you! If you haven't seen it, open your eyes and your mind. It's easy to remove those mental blinders and barriers, as long as you truly want to.

✧ Opportunities.

Seek out and you shall find opportunities to grow and connect with life without judging yourself. By staying in the moment with those who are nearest and dearest to us, we can cultivate compassion, love, kindness, and morality within us—and then extend this compassionate attitude towards others.

✧ Within.

By becoming more mindful, you will achieve a stronger inner peace. It is foremost beneficial to you, and then—from you—it explodes tenfold out into the world around you. You can be deeply affected by the people around you, and can gain insight from and power over their thoughts; never forget that this is mutual—so work to make a positive impact.

> "Mindfulness is simply being aware of what is happening right now without wishing it were different; enjoying the pleasant without holding on when it changes (which it will); being with the unpleasant without fearing it will always be this way (which it won't)." –James Baraz

THE PATH TO MINDFULNESS

Narcissists typically do not empathize nor can they appreciate the beauty of the life that surrounds them. They exist at the opposite end of the spectrum as opposed to compassion. John "woke up" when May died; this was the emotional event that triggered his realization—too late—that life extended beyond himself.

Mindfulness is about exactly that: waking up to the world and connecting with life.

As a teacher of mindfulness meditation and the founder of the University of Massachusetts's Mindfulness-Based Stress Reduction Program, Jon

Kabat-Zinn says: "Mindfulness means paying attention in a particular way; on purpose, in the present moment, and nonjudgmentally." By cultivating conscious awareness of the present moment, we extract ourselves from our own toxic thought patterns. By learning to sense and see and appreciate life, we need not regret an unfulfilled existence. Mindfulness is a practice that can immediately ground us back into the world, helping us delve within ourselves while simultaneously shifting us beyond ourselves.

PRACTICE

Not sure where to start? Dr. Kabat-Zinn lists the following simple exercises as key components to mastering mindfulness:

→ Pay attention to your breathing in the present moment.

→ Notice what you're sensing right now—use all of your senses. What can you see, hear, smell, touch, and taste? Increase your awareness of your body's physical sensations to better ground yourself in the moment.

→ Understand that your thoughts and emotions are like clouds. They will come and go and will always pass through; they need not define you.

→ Keep a look-out for negative thought patterns so that you recognize them and then can make changes.

Get out of your head and get into your soul. Don't waste life—*live it*. And begin living it now. If you do it now, you will always have time.

> "By breaking down our sense of self-importance, all we lose is a parasite that has long infected our minds. What we gain in return is freedom, openness of mind, spontaneity, simplicity, altruism: all qualities inherent in happiness." –Mathieu Ricard

USING MINDFULNESS TO BREAK THE CHAINS OF MENTAL SLAVERY

☑ *Do you sometimes feel suffocated by societal pressures or biases? Do you feel that you may have a different outlook that you've been stifling or ignoring?*

☑ *Do you feel isolated when you experience loss, rejection, or failure?*

☑ *Would you consider yourself a slave to your mind?*

PRISONER OF THE MIND

In her inspiring book, *The Invention of Wings*, Sue Monk Kidd examines themes of courage, hope, individuality, and the quest for freedom and self-discovery. The story is set in nineteenth-century Charleston, where an urban slave named Hetty "Handful" Grimke and the rich plantation owner's daughter, Sarah, come to realize that they are more similar than they thought. Although Handful is a slave—thus physically forced to work as ordered, and unable to leave the premises of the plantation without permission—it becomes apparent that Sarah is also imprisoned; she is enslaved by her own limiting and negative thoughts, hemmed in by

---

the limits imposed on her gender and status, and suffocated by social conditioning.

Handful makes the incisive observation about herself and Sarah. Handful notes that, though she is literally a prisoner of the plantation due to her slave status, Sarah lives in the prison of her own thoughts. At some point, Handful even tells Sarah: *"My body might be a slave, but not my mind. For you, it's the other way around."* As the story unfolds, Sarah discovers her voice after deep contemplation and self-reflection. Ultimately she is able to express herself and reveal her own true feelings about slavery. Over time, she discovers that her biases were imposed on her by society; accepting slavery was an act that actually goes against who she is and what she truly believes in.

> "You got to figure out which end of the needle you're gon' be, the one that's fastened to the thread or the end that pierces the cloth." –Sue Monk Kidd

NOW

Mindfulness is a universal and timeless tool that we can use to observe our ideas in the present moment without judgment. We can use mindfulness to choose the thoughts which express our deepest values of compassion for ourselves and others. We enable ourselves to grow and live more fully, discovering that hate consumes us but love expands our minds.

The NOW technique can enable us to do so.

✧ Notice.

Although Sarah was consciously repulsed by slavery, she was frozen by complacency. It wasn't until she could step back and examine her own thoughts that she began to live with integrity, conviction, and courage. It was only then that she could take positive action.

✧ Opportunities.

Just so, we can remain frozen in the past, ignoring our capabilities to notice and become curious about the roots of our problematic thoughts and behaviors. Or, we can choose to break free of these toxic chains and move forward. Acknowledging our behavior and attitude gives us the leverage to change them.

✧ Within.

Sarah was able to rewrite the direction of her thoughts—and thus her life—after she became consciously aware of the old, destructive thinking which she harbored within her mind. By changing her inner thoughts, she changed her outward behavior. She indeed became the change she wished to see in the world.

THE PATH TO MINDFULNESS

Research on mindfulness and self-compassion has proven time and time again that these practices lead toward healing and a sense of wholeness. As a practicing psychotherapist, I've seen many people over the decades whom I helped on their journey towards self-awareness. They became aware of deep-seated problems that were recurring and specifically triggered. They realized that they acted on subconscious thoughts that had been programmed into them and which they didn't genuinely believe in.

I recently dealt with a woman who was never able to allow herself to relax. This was taking a severe toll on her mental and physical health. She came to realize that the roots of her symptoms were deep and far-reaching, transmitted down through generations in her family. When I gently asked her if she believed that people should never be allowed to rest, she immediately began to shake her head. Her true belief didn't reflect her constant self-bias. Once she realized that, she began to ease free of her own mind trap.

PRACTICE

Dr. Kristin Neff, Associate Professor of Human Development at the University of Texas and self-proclaimed "pioneering self-compassion researcher", recommends a practice of Mindful Self-Compassion to help examine the roots of painful thoughts, feelings, and behaviors. For over a decade, she's been defining and measuring the construct. She's even developed workshops and programs, revolving around self-compassion, humanity and empathy, and mindfulness. Her self-compassion videos, in particular, walk you through:

→ **Self-Kindness**: Being kind, gentle, and understanding with yourself—as you would be to a friend—when you're suffering, in order to avoid shame, depression, and anxiety.

→ **Common Humanity**: Realizing that you're not alone in your struggles. When we're struggling, we tend to feel especially isolated. We suffer from the illusion that we're the worst—or that we're the only ones to experience loss, make mistakes, feel rejection, or fail.

→ **Mindfulness**: This is the practice of observing life as it is, without being judgmental or suppressing your thoughts and feelings.

It's important to relate *to* your thoughts and emotions—not to just turn away from or reject them outright. Develop a practice of noticing and labeling your emotions as they arise. For instance, when you are speaking with a person, you might notice that you are judging him; label those thoughts as *judgmental*. You may meet someone who intimidates you; notice that you are feeling fear in her presence, and label that feeling as *fear*. Being conscious in this manner will allow you to notice the thoughts which diminish you or others. Monitor what you believe and experience, and seek out opportunities to see yourself and the world with greater clarity and compassion.

"Today, like every other day, we wake up empty and frightened. Don't open the door to the study and begin reading. Take down a musical instrument." –Rumi

WASHING THE WINDOWS OF YOUR MIND'S EYE: INSIGHT FROM *A ROOM WITH A VIEW*

☑ *Do you struggle with addiction?*

☑ *Do you feel overwhelmed by destructive habits?*

☑ *Do you wish that you could make healthier decisions?*

A DIFFERENT PERSPECTIVE

In his internationally acclaimed novel *A Room With a View*, author E. M. Forster brushes upon themes of identity, self-transformation and growth, love, hypocrisy, and societal boundaries, among other things. His heroine, a spirited young woman named Lucy, grapples with a personal identity crisis. She is torn between the constraining expectations of her conventional, conservative, Edwardian England upbringing and the lure of a more independent, questioning, adventurous state of being that is triggered by her travels and experiences.

Forster delves deeper to reveal another outlook on identity: that "home" is a place we carry within us, and that it is we who create the world around us through our own eyes: *"We cast a shadow on something wherever we stand,*

and it is no good moving from place to place to save things; because the shadow always follows. Choose a place where you won't do harm—yes, choose a place where you won't do very much harm, and stand in it for all you are worth, facing the sunshine."

It appears, then, that not only is home a place you carry within you, yet that your issues and joys and ordeals are also things you carry in your inner world and magnify in your mind's eye.

These issues include addictions.

> "Our own worst enemy cannot harm us as much as our unwise thoughts. No one can help us as much as our own compassionate thoughts." –Buddha

NOW

While context changes a situation, it is ultimately up to us to decide how we interpret and use this context. My own Scottish ancestors, for instance, survived the infamous Potato Famine. After living through the famine, they carried with them an appreciation and craving for foods that they had been deprived of during those difficult days. They'd allowed the famine to significantly affect their outlook on food, and they passed down this mentality to later generations. Their descendants were farmers who also experienced droughts and pests that endangered their food supplies; they could relate very strongly to that old mentality.

As a child—with a child's malleable mind—I was fed these stories of hunger and was taught the value of food. Leaving food on a plate was sacrilege. Foods that my ancestors used to dream about—fried foods, vegetables prepared with bacon grease, and sweet tea loaded with syrupy sugar—were "precious", not "unhealthy"; so, the more the better. My ancestors' perceptions were handed down to me, and I stuck with those old beliefs even though they didn't make sense in the new context—*my* context, where food was plentiful, my body couldn't burn off extra calories and instead stored them as excess fat, and I had the privilege of choosing my meals and being educated about healthy nourishment.

I began to incorporate the NOW approach in my attitude towards food:

❖ Notice.

I first had to become aware of the unhealthy messages I was receiving about food. If I maintained the mindset of my starving ancestors ("eat as much as possible while and whenever you can—because you'll very rarely get this chance—and eat fatty foods to sustain yourself for longer") who lived in a very different situation, I would be killing myself instead of saving myself. Instead of putting some meat on my bones, I'd be at risk for obesity, heart disease, cholesterol, blood pressure, blood sugar spikes, acne, insulin resistance, and a heap of other life-threatening problems.

❖ Opportunities.

I had to notice how I felt in these situations. When I overate or ate unhealthy foods, I had the opportunity to see how my body negatively reacted. When I began to follow a more healthy diet and regime, I was astounded at how wonderful and energized I began to feel over time. I always tried to pay close attention to what my body was telling me.

❖ Within.

The third and final step of the process is about consciously deciding to develop different habits. You understand the need and thus you decide to change. Each day unravels as a series of choices to incorporate healthier habits and behaviors that will eventually streamline into a new and better lifestyle.

"If we are unaware of our present actions, we are condemned to repeating the mistakes of the past. But if we can develop the ability to be aware of the present moment, we can use the past as a guide for ordering our actions in the

future, so that we may attain our goal." –S. N.
Goenka

THE PATH TO MINDFULNESS

My prevailing subconscious thoughts were that those unhealthy foods were valuable and demanded appreciation. It was challenging for me to become conscious of the misaligned messages that I'd received about food. To be healthy, however, I realized that I had to learn to realign my perspective and make healthier choices.

When you are grappling with an addiction or a destructive behavior, just remember to take a step back and explore the issue. Note—without judgement—what is really going on and where this mentality is coming from. Figure out why this lifestyle harms instead of helps you, and seek out a better alternative. Discover what the best solution is and work towards that. Decide to make those new habits a new lifestyle.

Remember that, regardless of how you choose to describe the journey (life is about finding yourself; life is about creating yourself), the fact remains that *you* are in charge of its direction.

PRACTICE

Ask yourself:

→ What do I believe about this habit/behavior? What is my mentality?

→ When did I first learn this? Who taught me? What was the backstory?

→ How does their story align with mine? How do the contexts differ? Is this something that doesn't align or make sense anymore? (Remember your brain is always trying to protect you—you learn behaviors for a reason.)

→ How could I rewrite this story/mentality to benefit me? What habits would I change? What changes would come of this?

Incorporate these changes and notice the difference. How does the new behavior make you feel? Does it make sense? You should be able to see the purpose and potential of this. Will this help? I promise that it will. Immensely.

Mindfulness helped me transform my outlook and my habits—and thus my life. I realized what translated as "survival" for my ancestors didn't equate to "survival" for me (it meant the opposite!). Like Lucy in *A Room With a View*, I realized that I'd have to pick up the pen and write out my own destiny—or else others would write it for me. I learned what "survival" and "health" and "well-being" meant *for me,* personally, and then that's what I pursued. My new habits became a lifestyle.

My body thanks me for those choices every day by keeping me healthy.

> "Between stimulus and response there is a space. In that space is our power to create our response. In our response lies our growth and our freedom." –Viktor Frankl

CONCLUSION

Remember that the stories in this book are designed to be reread as reminders at any time during your life's journey. They're always available to offer you a glimpse into the trials and triumphs of others, into the real-world use and benefits of mindfulness, and into the simple yet life-altering ways by which you can incorporate mindfulness into your own life from this very moment. They are here to remind you, my friend, that you are not alone—that you've never been alone.

You can program your incredible human brain. Only you can decide to make the shift from judgmental thinking, toxic people, and negativity. By exploring avenues of living more fully in the moment, by practicing loving kindness, and by exuding gratitude for the abundance that surrounds you, you have the capability to break down any mental barriers that keep you from living life mindfully and joyfully. Shed the toxins and unleash your pure, true self.

If you do it now, you will always have time.

INDEX

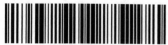

Made in the USA
San Bernardino, CA
13 November 2016